KIDNEY DISEASE DIET COOKBOOK FOR WOMEN

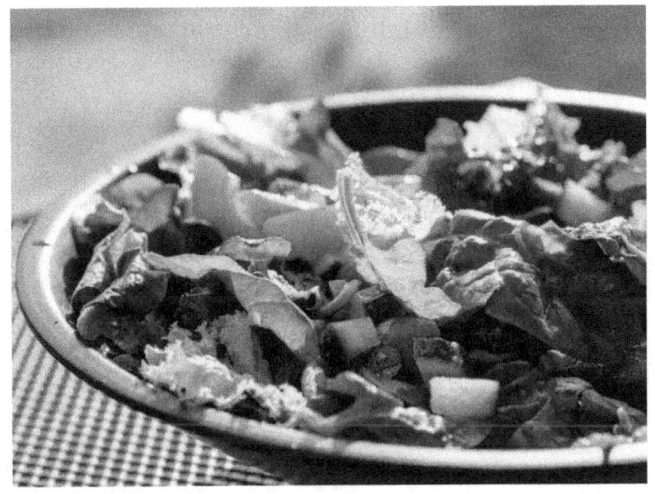

DR. JESSICA SMITH

Copyright © 2024 by DR. JESSICA SMITH

All rights reserved.

No part of this book may be reproduced, stored in a retrieval system, or transmitted, in any form or by any means, electronic, mechanical, photocopying, recording, or otherwise, without prior written permission from the publisher, except for brief quotations embodied in critical articles or reviews.

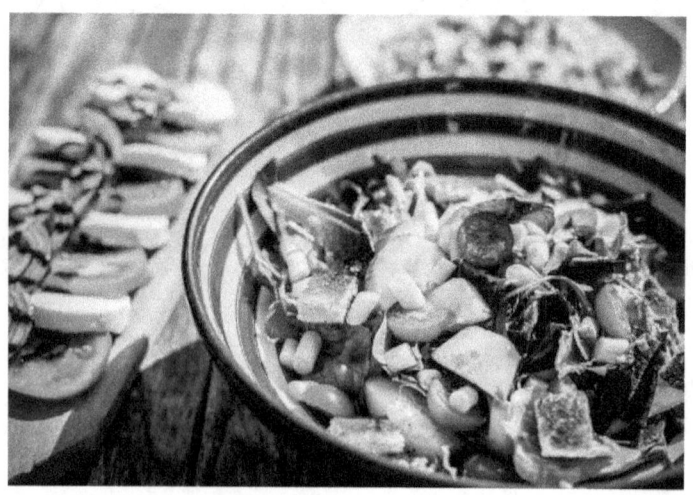

TABLE OF CONTENTS

CHAPTER ONE 7

How to Use this Cookbook 7

Understanding Kidney Disease Diet for Women 9

Benefits of Kidney Disease Diet for Women ... 11

Guidelines for Kidney Disease Diet for Women 12

Causes of Kidney Disease in Women 14

Types of Kidney Disease in Women 16

Symptoms of kidney disease in Women 18

Risk Factor of Kidney Disease in Women 20

CHAPTER TWO 23

Kidney Disease Breakfast Recipes for Women 23

1: Vegetable Omelette 23

2: Berry and Yogurt Parfait 25

3: Quinoa Breakfast Bowl 26

4: Avocado Toast with Poached Egg 28

5: Spinach and Mushroom Breakfast Wrap 29

6: Chia Seed Pudding 31

7: Overnight Oats with Berries 33

8: Green Smoothie 34

9: Veggie Breakfast Burrito 36

10: Cottage Cheese and Fruit Bowl 38

Kidney Disease Lunch Recipes for Women 39

1: Quinoa Salad with Chickpeas and Veggies .. 39

2: Salmon and Avocado Wrap 41

3: Turkey and Vegetable Stir-Fry 43

4: Lentil and Vegetable Soup 45

5: Chicken and Quinoa Salad 47

6: Tuna Salad Stuffed Bell Peppers 49

7: Mediterranean Chickpea Salad 51

8: Veggie and Hummus Wrap 53

9: Veggie and Bean Quesadillas 55

10: Spinach and Lentil Salad 57

Kidney Disease Dinner Recipes for Women 59

1: Baked Salmon with Asparagus 59

2: Turkey and Vegetable Stir-Fry 61

3: Veggie and Lentil Soup 63

4: Grilled Chicken with Roasted Vegetables 65

5: Quinoa Stuffed Bell Peppers 67

6: Veggie Stir-Fry with Tofu 70

7: Mediterranean Chicken Skewers with Greek Salad 72

8: Lentil and Vegetable Curry 75

9: Baked Cod with Lemon Herb Crust 77

10: Turkey Meatballs with Marinara Sauce 79

Kidney Disease Snacks Recipes for Women 82

1: Avocado and White Bean Dip with Veggie Sticks..82

2: Greek Yogurt Parfait with Berries and Almonds...84

3: Hummus with Whole Grain Pita Chips........86

4: Cottage Cheese with Sliced Peaches and Almonds...88

5: Tuna Salad Stuffed Cucumber Boats............90

6: Rice Cake with Almond Butter and Banana Slices..91

7: Edamame Hummus with Raw Veggie Dippers 93

8: Apple Slices with Peanut Butter and Chia Seeds..95

9: Cucumber and Cottage Cheese Bites 96

10: Banana and Walnut Oat Bites.....................98

CONCLUSION 101

CHAPTER ONE

How to Use this Cookbook

Understand Your Dietary Restrictions: Start by understanding the dietary restrictions associated with kidney disease. This typically includes limitations on sodium, potassium, phosphorus, and protein intake.

Read the Introduction: Take the time to read the introduction of the cookbook. It usually contains valuable information about kidney health, dietary guidelines, and how to use the cookbook effectively.

Consult with a Dietitian: If possible, consult with a registered dietitian specializing in kidney health. They can help you understand your specific dietary needs and how to adapt recipes accordingly.

Plan Your Meals: Use the cookbook to plan your meals for the week. Look for recipes that align with your dietary requirements and preferences.

Check Ingredients and Nutritional Information: Before starting any recipe, carefully check the ingredients and nutritional information provided in the cookbook.

Pay attention to portion sizes and any substitutions recommended for kidney-friendly options.

Prepare Your Kitchen: Make sure your kitchen is stocked with kidney-friendly ingredients such as fresh fruits, vegetables, lean proteins, and whole grains. Organize your cooking utensils and tools for easy access.

Follow Recipes Carefully: Follow the recipes in the cookbook step by step, ensuring you measure ingredients accurately. This helps maintain the appropriate balance of nutrients and flavors.

Experiment with Flavors: Don't be afraid to experiment with herbs, spices, and low-sodium seasonings to enhance the flavor of your dishes without compromising your kidney health.

Listen to Your Body: Pay attention to how your body responds to different meals. Keep track of your symptoms and energy levels. Adjust your diet as needed and consult with your healthcare team if you have any concerns.

Remember, consistency and moderation are key when following a kidney disease diet.

With the right resources and support, you can enjoy delicious and nutritious meals while managing your kidney health effectively.

Understanding Kidney Disease Diet for Women

Understanding the kidney disease diet for women is crucial for managing the condition effectively.

Women with kidney disease often face unique challenges due to factors such as hormonal fluctuations and differences in body composition.

The primary goals of the kidney disease diet for women are to preserve kidney function, manage symptoms, and prevent complications.

Central to this dietary approach is controlling intake of certain nutrients, including sodium, potassium, phosphorus, and protein.

Sodium restriction is important for managing blood pressure and fluid balance, while controlling potassium and phosphorus helps prevent electrolyte imbalances and mineral buildup in the bloodstream.

Protein intake may be moderated to reduce strain on the kidneys while still meeting nutritional needs.

Additionally, women with kidney disease may need to pay attention to their calcium and vitamin D intake to support bone health, as kidney dysfunction can affect the body's ability to regulate these nutrients.

A kidney disease diet for women typically emphasizes whole, nutrient-rich foods such as fruits, vegetables, whole grains, and lean proteins.

Portion control and meal planning are essential strategies for maintaining nutritional balance while adhering to dietary restrictions.

Consulting with a registered dietitian who specializes in kidney health can provide personalized guidance and support.

By understanding and adhering to the kidney disease diet for women, individuals can help manage their condition and improve overall quality of life.

Benefits of Kidney Disease Diet for Women

The kidney disease diet offers several benefits specifically tailored to women, helping them manage their condition effectively and improve overall health outcomes.

One significant advantage is the ability to control blood pressure. Many women with kidney disease also experience hypertension, which can exacerbate kidney damage and increase the risk of cardiovascular complications.

By reducing sodium intake and adhering to a kidney-friendly diet, women can help regulate blood pressure levels, reducing strain on the kidneys and lowering the risk of further damage.

Another key benefit of the kidney disease diet for women is the ability to manage electrolyte balance. Potassium and phosphorus levels need to be closely monitored in individuals with kidney disease to prevent complications such as hyperkalemia and hyperphosphatemia.

By following dietary guidelines that limit these minerals, women can reduce the risk of electrolyte imbalances and associated symptoms like muscle weakness and bone disorders.

Additionally, the kidney disease diet promotes overall nutritional wellness.

By focusing on whole, nutrient-rich foods and controlling portion sizes, women can ensure they are meeting their dietary needs while minimizing the intake of substances that may worsen kidney function.

This balanced approach supports overall health and well-being, helping women with kidney disease feel their best and maintain a higher quality of life.

Guidelines for Kidney Disease Diet for Women

The kidney disease diet for women follows specific guidelines aimed at preserving kidney function, managing symptoms, and preventing complications.

These guidelines focus on controlling intake of certain nutrients while promoting overall nutritional balance:

Limit Sodium: Women with kidney disease should reduce their sodium intake to help manage blood pressure and fluid balance. This involves avoiding high-sodium processed foods and using alternative seasonings to flavor meals.

Monitor Potassium and Phosphorus: Potassium and phosphorus levels must be closely monitored to prevent electrolyte imbalances. Women should limit foods high in these minerals, such as bananas, oranges, tomatoes (potassium), and dairy products, nuts, and seeds (phosphorus).

Moderate Protein Intake: While protein is essential for overall health, consuming too much can put strain on the kidneys. Women with kidney disease may need to moderate their protein intake, opting for lean sources such as poultry, fish, and plant-based proteins.

Control Fluid Intake: Individuals with kidney disease may need to limit their fluid intake to avoid fluid overload and swelling. Women should monitor their fluid intake, including beverages and foods with high water content.

Focus on Nutrient-Rich Foods: The kidney disease diet encourages consumption of nutrient-rich foods such as fruits, vegetables, whole grains, and lean proteins to meet nutritional needs while minimizing the intake of processed foods and added sugars.

Work with a Dietitian: Consulting with a registered dietitian who specializes in kidney health can provide personalized guidance and support in adhering to dietary guidelines and making appropriate food choices.

Causes of Kidney Disease in Women

Kidney disease in women can arise from a variety of causes, some of which may be unique to female physiology and health conditions.

Understanding these causes is crucial for prevention, early detection, and effective management:

Autoimmune Diseases: Certain autoimmune diseases like lupus and rheumatoid arthritis are more common in women and can lead to kidney inflammation (glomerulonephritis) and damage over time.

Urinary Tract Infections (UTIs): Women are more prone to UTIs due to their shorter urethra, which allows bacteria easier access to the bladder and kidneys. Recurrent or untreated UTIs can lead to kidney infections and damage.

Pregnancy-Related Complications: Pregnancy can put strain on the kidneys, leading to conditions like preeclampsia or gestational diabetes, which may cause kidney damage if not managed properly.

High Blood Pressure (Hypertension): Hypertension is a leading cause of kidney disease in both men and women. Women, particularly as they age, may be more susceptible to hypertension, especially if they have hormonal imbalances or are postmenopausal.

Diabetes: Women with diabetes are at increased risk of developing kidney disease. Diabetes can damage the small blood vessels in the kidneys over time, leading to impaired kidney function or kidney failure.

Chronic Urinary Tract Obstruction: Conditions such as kidney stones or congenital abnormalities in the urinary tract can cause chronic obstruction, leading to kidney damage over time.

Medications and Toxins: Certain medications, especially when used long-term, and exposure to toxins can damage the kidneys. Women may be more susceptible due to differences in medication metabolism and toxin exposure.

By understanding these potential causes, women can take proactive steps to reduce their risk of kidney disease through lifestyle modifications, regular health screenings, and appropriate management of underlying health conditions.

Early detection and intervention are key to preserving kidney function and overall health.

Types of Kidney Disease in Women

Kidney disease encompasses a range of conditions that affect the structure and function of the kidneys.

While many types of kidney disease can affect both men and women, some may have specific implications for women due to hormonal factors or pregnancy.

Here are several types of kidney disease that commonly affect women:

Chronic Kidney Disease (CKD): CKD is a progressive condition where the kidneys gradually lose function over time. Women with CKD may experience complications related to hormonal changes, such as bone loss or menstrual irregularities.

Glomerulonephritis: This is a group of diseases that cause inflammation and damage to the glomeruli, the tiny filters in the kidneys.

Lupus nephritis, a type of glomerulonephritis, is more common in women and is associated with the autoimmune disease lupus.

Polycystic Kidney Disease (PKD): PKD is a genetic disorder characterized by the growth of cysts in the kidneys. While PKD affects both men and women, women with PKD may experience additional complications during pregnancy due to the increased strain on the kidneys.

Urinary Tract Infections (UTIs): UTIs are more common in women due to their shorter urethra, which allows bacteria easier access to the bladder and kidneys. Recurrent or untreated UTIs can lead to kidney infections and damage.

Kidney Stones: While kidney stones can affect anyone, women may be more susceptible to certain types of stones due to hormonal factors. Pregnancy and hormonal birth control methods can also increase the risk of developing kidney stones in women.

Understanding the different types of kidney disease that affect women is essential for early detection, proper management, and prevention of complications. Regular health screenings, lifestyle modifications, and management of underlying health conditions are key to maintaining kidney health in women.

Symptoms of kidney disease in Women

Symptoms of kidney disease in women can vary depending on the underlying cause and the stage of the condition.

Early stages of kidney disease may not present noticeable symptoms, making regular health check-ups and screenings crucial for early detection.

However, as kidney function declines, various symptoms may manifest, including:

Changes in Urination: Women with kidney disease may experience changes in urination patterns, such as increased frequency, foamy urine, or blood in the urine (hematuria). They may also experience difficulty urinating or have to urinate during the night (nocturia).

Swelling: Kidney dysfunction can lead to fluid retention, resulting in swelling in the ankles, feet, hands, or face. This swelling, known as edema, occurs due to the kidneys' inability to properly regulate fluid balance and may worsen throughout the day.

Fatigue and Weakness: Decreased kidney function can lead to the accumulation of toxins and waste products in the body, resulting in fatigue, weakness, and overall lethargy.

Shortness of Breath: As kidney disease progresses, excess fluid buildup in the lungs can cause shortness of breath, particularly during physical activity or when lying down.

High Blood Pressure: Hypertension (high blood pressure) is both a cause and a symptom of kidney disease. Women with kidney disease may experience elevated blood pressure, which can further damage the kidneys if left uncontrolled.

Nausea and Vomiting: Buildup of waste products in the bloodstream can lead to nausea, vomiting, loss of appetite, and weight loss.

Bone Pain and Weakness: Kidney disease can affect bone health, leading to bone pain, weakness, and an increased risk of fractures due to abnormalities in calcium and phosphorus metabolism.

Early intervention can help slow the progression of the disease and prevent complications.

Risk Factor of Kidney Disease in Women

Kidney disease poses a significant health risk to women, with various factors contributing to its development and progression.

Understanding these risk factors is crucial for prevention, early detection, and effective management. Some key risk factors of kidney disease in women include:

Diabetes: Women with diabetes are at a higher risk of developing kidney disease compared to those without diabetes. Prolonged high blood sugar levels can damage the small blood vessels in the kidneys, leading to diabetic nephropathy and impaired kidney function.

High Blood Pressure (Hypertension): Hypertension is a leading cause of kidney disease in both men and women. Women, particularly as they age, may be more susceptible to hypertension, especially if they have hormonal imbalances or are postmenopausal.

Autoimmune Diseases: Conditions such as lupus and rheumatoid arthritis are more prevalent in women and can lead to kidney inflammation (glomerulonephritis) and damage over time.

Urinary Tract Infections (UTIs): Women are more prone to UTIs due to their shorter urethra, which allows bacteria easier access to the bladder and kidneys. Recurrent or untreated UTIs can lead to kidney infections and damage.

Obesity: Excess weight, particularly abdominal fat, is associated with an increased risk of kidney disease in women. Obesity can contribute to insulin resistance, hypertension, and other metabolic abnormalities that can damage the kidneys over time.

Family History: Women with a family history of kidney disease are at a higher risk of developing the condition themselves. Genetic factors can predispose individuals to certain kidney diseases, such as polycystic kidney disease (PKD).

Pregnancy-Related Complications: Certain pregnancy-related complications, such as preeclampsia or gestational diabetes, can increase the risk of kidney disease in women, especially if left untreated or poorly managed.

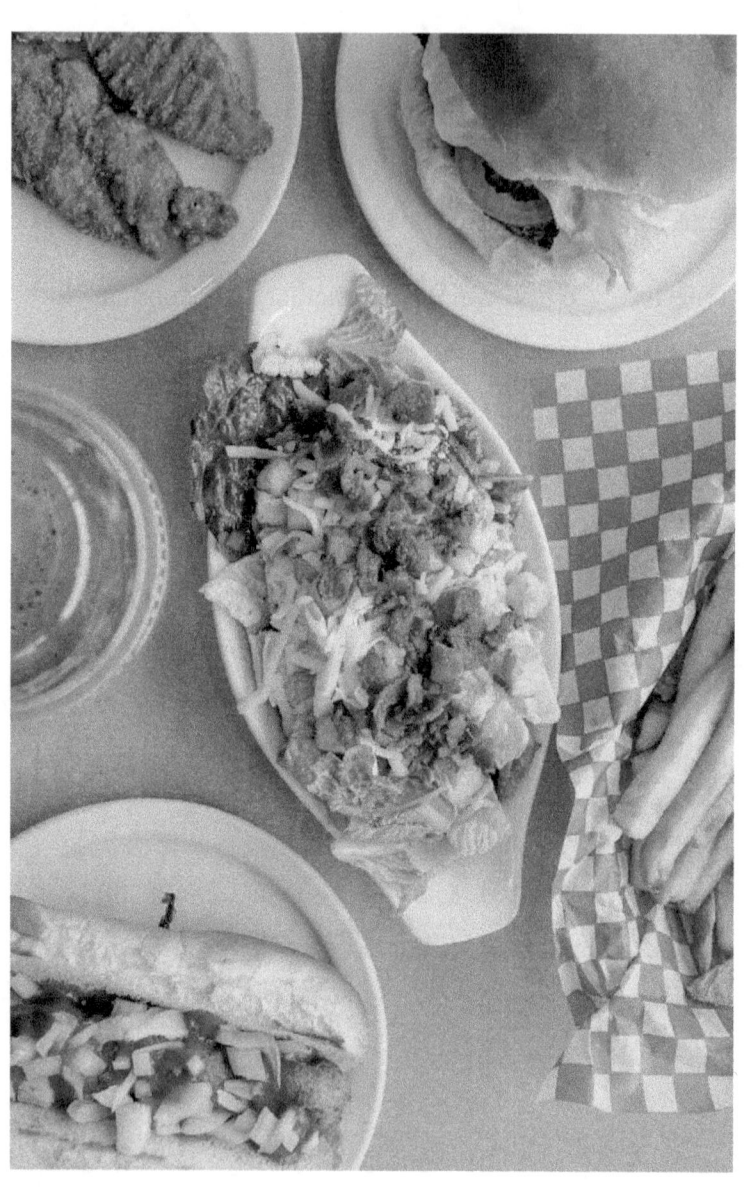

CHAPTER TWO

Kidney Disease Breakfast Recipes for Women

1: Vegetable Omelette

Ingredients:

- 2 eggs
- 1/4 cup diced bell peppers (any color)
- 1/4 cup diced onions
- 1/4 cup chopped spinach
- 1 tablespoon olive oil
- Salt and pepper to taste

Instructions:

- In a bowl, beat the eggs and season with salt and pepper.
- Heat olive oil in a non-stick skillet over medium heat.
- Add the diced bell peppers and onions to the skillet and sauté until softened, about 2-3 minutes.
- Add the chopped spinach to the skillet and cook for another 1-2 minutes until wilted.

- Pour the beaten eggs over the vegetables in the skillet, tilting the pan to spread them evenly.
- Cook the omelette for 2-3 minutes until the edges start to set.
- Using a spatula, gently lift the edges of the omelette and tilt the skillet to let the uncooked eggs flow underneath.
- Once the omelette is mostly set, fold it in half and cook for another 1-2 minutes until cooked through.
- Slide the omelette onto a plate and serve hot.

Health Benefits:

- This vegetable omelette is rich in protein from the eggs, which is essential for muscle health and satiety.
- The bell peppers and spinach provide vitamins, minerals, and antioxidants that support overall health and immune function.
- Olive oil adds healthy fats, which are beneficial for heart health and nutrient absorption.

Preparation Time: 10 minutes

2: Berry and Yogurt Parfait

Ingredients:

- 1/2 cup plain Greek yogurt
- 1/4 cup mixed berries (such as strawberries, blueberries, and raspberries)
- 2 tablespoons chopped nuts (such as almonds or walnuts)
- 1 tablespoon honey or maple syrup (optional)

Instructions:

- In a glass or bowl, layer half of the Greek yogurt.
- Add half of the mixed berries on top of the yogurt layer.
- Sprinkle half of the chopped nuts over the berries.
- Repeat the layers with the remaining yogurt, berries, and nuts.
- Drizzle honey or maple syrup on top if desired.
- Serve immediately or refrigerate until ready to eat.

Health Benefits:

- Greek yogurt is a good source of protein and probiotics, which support digestive health and immunity.
- Berries are rich in antioxidants, vitamins, and fiber, which promote heart health, brain function, and weight management.
- Nuts provide healthy fats, protein, and essential nutrients like vitamin E and magnesium, which are beneficial for overall health.

Preparation Time: 5 minutes

3: Quinoa Breakfast Bowl

Ingredients:

- 1/2 cup cooked quinoa
- 1/4 cup sliced strawberries
- 1/4 cup diced mango
- 2 tablespoons chopped almonds
- 1 tablespoon honey or maple syrup (optional)
- 1/4 teaspoon cinnamon

Instructions:

- In a bowl, combine the cooked quinoa, sliced strawberries, diced mango, and chopped almonds.
- Drizzle honey or maple syrup over the mixture if desired.
- Sprinkle cinnamon on top for added flavor.
- Stir gently to combine all the ingredients.
- Serve immediately as a warm breakfast bowl or chill in the refrigerator for a refreshing breakfast option.

Health Benefits:

- Quinoa is a high-protein grain that provides essential amino acids, fiber, and minerals like iron and magnesium, supporting muscle health and energy levels.
- Strawberries and mangoes are rich in vitamins, antioxidants, and fiber, which promote heart health, immune function, and digestion.
- Almonds offer healthy fats, protein, and vitamin E, contributing to heart health and satiety.

Preparation Time: 15 minutes

4: Avocado Toast with Poached Egg

Ingredients:

- 1 slice whole-grain bread
- 1/2 ripe avocado, mashed
- 1 poached egg
- Salt and pepper to taste
- Red pepper flakes (optional)
- Fresh parsley or cilantro for garnish (optional)

Instructions:

- Toast the whole-grain bread until golden brown.
- Spread the mashed avocado evenly on top of the toast.
- Carefully place the poached egg on top of the mashed avocado.
- Season with salt, pepper, and red pepper flakes if desired.
- Garnish with fresh parsley or cilantro for added flavor and presentation.
- Serve immediately while the poached egg is still warm.

Health Benefits:

- Whole-grain bread provides fiber, vitamins, and minerals, promoting digestive health and steady energy levels.
- Avocado is rich in healthy fats, fiber, and potassium, supporting heart health and satiety.
- Poached eggs offer high-quality protein and essential nutrients like vitamin D and B vitamins, contributing to muscle health and overall well-being.

Preparation Time: 10 minutes

5: Spinach and Mushroom Breakfast Wrap

Ingredients:

- 1 whole-wheat tortilla
- 2 large eggs
- 1/4 cup sliced mushrooms
- 1/4 cup chopped spinach
- 1 tablespoon olive oil
- Salt and pepper to taste
- 2 tablespoons shredded low-fat cheese (optional)

Instructions:

- Heat olive oil in a skillet over medium heat.
- Add sliced mushrooms to the skillet and sauté until golden brown, about 2-3 minutes.
- Add chopped spinach to the skillet and cook until wilted, about 1-2 minutes.
- In a separate bowl, beat the eggs and season with salt and pepper.
- Pour the beaten eggs into the skillet with the mushrooms and spinach.
- Cook the eggs, stirring occasionally, until they are scrambled and cooked through.
- Warm the whole-wheat tortilla in the microwave or on a skillet.
- Place the scrambled eggs, mushrooms, and spinach in the center of the tortilla.
- Optional: Sprinkle shredded low-fat cheese on top.
- Fold the sides of the tortilla over the filling to form a wrap.
- Serve immediately.

Health Benefits:

- Spinach and mushrooms provide vitamins, minerals, and antioxidants that support immune function and overall health.
- Whole-wheat tortillas offer fiber and complex carbohydrates for sustained energy levels.
- Eggs are a good source of protein and essential nutrients, promoting muscle health and satiety.

Preparation Time: 15 minutes

6: Chia Seed Pudding

Ingredients:

- 2 tablespoons chia seeds
- 1/2 cup unsweetened almond milk (or any milk of choice)
- 1/4 teaspoon vanilla extract
- 1 tablespoon honey or maple syrup (optional)
- Fresh fruit for topping (such as berries or sliced bananas)

Instructions:

- In a bowl, combine chia seeds, almond milk, vanilla extract, and honey or maple syrup (if using).
- Stir well to combine all ingredients.
- Cover the bowl and refrigerate for at least 2 hours or overnight, allowing the chia seeds to absorb the liquid and thicken into a pudding-like consistency.
- Once the chia seed pudding has set, give it a good stir.
- Transfer the pudding to a serving bowl or individual jars.
- Top with fresh fruit of your choice.
- Serve chilled.

Health Benefits:

- Chia seeds are rich in fiber, omega-3 fatty acids, and antioxidants, supporting digestive health, heart health, and inflammation reduction.
- Almond milk is low in calories and provides essential nutrients like vitamin E and calcium, promoting bone health and overall well-being.

- Fresh fruit offers vitamins, minerals, and fiber, contributing to hydration, immune function, and digestive health.

Preparation Time: 5 minutes (plus chilling time)

7: Overnight Oats with Berries

Ingredients:

- 1/2 cup rolled oats
- 1/2 cup unsweetened almond milk (or any milk of choice)
- 1/4 cup Greek yogurt
- 1/4 teaspoon vanilla extract
- 1 tablespoon honey or maple syrup (optional)
- 1/4 cup mixed berries (such as strawberries, blueberries, and raspberries)
- 1 tablespoon chopped nuts (such as almonds or walnuts)

Instructions:

- In a jar or bowl, combine rolled oats, almond milk, Greek yogurt, vanilla extract, and honey or maple syrup (if using). Stir well to combine.

- Add the mixed berries on top of the oat mixture.
- Cover the jar or bowl and refrigerate overnight, allowing the oats to absorb the liquid and soften.
- In the morning, give the oats a good stir.
- Top with chopped nuts for added crunch and flavor.
- Serve chilled.

Health Benefits:

- Rolled oats are a good source of fiber, providing sustained energy and promoting digestive health.
- Greek yogurt adds protein and probiotics, supporting muscle health and gut health.
- Berries are rich in antioxidants, vitamins, and fiber, offering numerous health benefits including improved heart health and cognitive function.

Preparation Time: 5 minutes (plus overnight chilling)

8: Green Smoothie

Ingredients:

- 1 cup fresh spinach leaves
- 1/2 ripe banana

- 1/2 cup frozen mixed berries (such as strawberries, blueberries, and raspberries)
- 1/2 cup unsweetened almond milk (or any milk of choice)
- 1 tablespoon chia seeds
- 1 tablespoon honey or maple syrup (optional)

Instructions:

- In a blender, combine fresh spinach leaves, banana, frozen mixed berries, almond milk, chia seeds, and honey or maple syrup (if using).
- Blend until smooth and creamy, adding more almond milk if needed to reach the desired consistency.
- Pour the smoothie into a glass.
- Optional: Garnish with additional berries or a sprinkle of chia seeds on top.
- Serve immediately.

Health Benefits:

- Spinach is rich in vitamins, minerals, and antioxidants, supporting immune function and overall health.

- Berries provide a burst of flavor and numerous health benefits including improved heart health and cognitive function.
- Chia seeds offer fiber, omega-3 fatty acids, and protein, promoting digestive health, heart health, and satiety.

Preparation Time: 5 minutes

9: Veggie Breakfast Burrito

Ingredients:

- 1 whole-grain tortilla
- 2 eggs, scrambled
- 1/4 cup diced bell peppers (any color)
- 1/4 cup diced tomatoes
- 2 tablespoons diced onions
- 2 tablespoons shredded low-fat cheese (optional)
- 1 tablespoon chopped cilantro (optional)
- Salt and pepper to taste
- Salsa or hot sauce (optional, for serving)

Instructions:

- Heat a non-stick skillet over medium heat.

- Add diced bell peppers, tomatoes, and onions to the skillet and sauté until softened, about 2-3 minutes.
- Remove the vegetables from the skillet and set aside.
- In the same skillet, add the scrambled eggs and cook until they are set, stirring occasionally.
- Warm the whole-grain tortilla in the microwave or on a skillet.
- Place the scrambled eggs and sautéed vegetables in the center of the tortilla.
- Optional: Sprinkle shredded low-fat cheese and chopped cilantro on top.
- Season with salt and pepper to taste.
- Fold the sides of the tortilla over the filling to form a burrito.
- Serve with salsa or hot sauce on the side if desired.

Health Benefits:

- Whole-grain tortillas provide fiber and complex carbohydrates for sustained energy levels.
- Eggs offer high-quality protein and essential nutrients, promoting muscle health and satiety.

- Bell peppers, tomatoes, onions, and cilantro are rich in vitamins, minerals, and antioxidants, supporting immune function and overall health.

Preparation Time: 10 minutes

10: Cottage Cheese and Fruit Bowl

Ingredients:

- 1/2 cup low-fat cottage cheese
- 1/2 cup mixed fresh fruit (such as pineapple chunks, peach slices, and kiwi)
- 1 tablespoon chopped nuts (such as almonds or walnuts)
- 1 teaspoon honey or maple syrup (optional)
- 1 tablespoon unsweetened coconut flakes (optional)

Instructions:

- In a bowl, scoop the low-fat cottage cheese.
- Top with mixed fresh fruit.
- Sprinkle chopped nuts over the fruit.
- Drizzle honey or maple syrup on top if desired.
- Optional: Garnish with unsweetened coconut flakes for added flavor.

- Serve immediately.

Health Benefits:

- Low-fat cottage cheese is a good source of protein and calcium, supporting muscle health and bone health.
- Fresh fruit offers vitamins, minerals, and antioxidants, promoting immune function, heart health, and digestion.
- Nuts provide healthy fats, protein, and essential nutrients, contributing to heart health, satiety, and overall well-being.

Preparation Time: 5 minutes

Kidney Disease Lunch Recipes for Women

1: Quinoa Salad with Chickpeas and Veggies

Ingredients:

- 1/2 cup cooked quinoa
- 1/2 cup canned chickpeas, rinsed and drained
- 1/4 cup diced cucumber
- 1/4 cup diced bell peppers (any color)
- 1/4 cup cherry tomatoes, halved

- 2 tablespoons chopped fresh parsley
- 1 tablespoon olive oil
- 1 tablespoon lemon juice
- Salt and pepper to taste
- Optional: crumbled feta cheese

Instructions:

- In a large bowl, combine cooked quinoa, chickpeas, diced cucumber, diced bell peppers, cherry tomatoes, and chopped parsley.
- In a small bowl, whisk together olive oil, lemon juice, salt, and pepper to make the dressing.
- Pour the dressing over the quinoa salad and toss to coat evenly.
- Optional: Sprinkle crumbled feta cheese on top for added flavor.
- Serve immediately or refrigerate until ready to eat.

Health Benefits:

- Quinoa is a complete protein and a good source of fiber, supporting muscle health and digestion.

- Chickpeas provide protein and fiber, promoting satiety and digestive health.
- Vegetables like cucumber, bell peppers, and cherry tomatoes are rich in vitamins, minerals, and antioxidants, supporting immune function and overall health.
- Olive oil offers heart-healthy fats and anti-inflammatory properties, contributing to cardiovascular health.

Preparation Time: 15 minutes

2: Salmon and Avocado Wrap

Ingredients:

- 1 whole-grain tortilla
- 3 oz cooked salmon, flaked
- 1/4 ripe avocado, sliced
- 1/4 cup shredded lettuce
- 2 tablespoons diced tomatoes
- 1 tablespoon Greek yogurt
- 1 teaspoon Dijon mustard
- Salt and pepper to taste

Instructions:

- Lay the whole-grain tortilla flat on a plate or cutting board.
- Spread Greek yogurt and Dijon mustard evenly over the tortilla.
- Layer shredded lettuce, flaked salmon, sliced avocado, and diced tomatoes on top of the tortilla.
- Season with salt and pepper to taste.
- Roll up the tortilla tightly to form a wrap.
- Optional: Secure the wrap with toothpicks or cut it in half for easier handling.
- Serve immediately or pack it for a convenient on-the-go lunch.

Health Benefits:

- Salmon is rich in omega-3 fatty acids, protein, and vitamin D, supporting heart health, brain function, and bone health.
- Avocado offers healthy fats, fiber, and potassium, promoting heart health and satiety.

- Whole-grain tortillas provide fiber and complex carbohydrates for sustained energy levels and digestive health.
- Greek yogurt adds protein and probiotics, supporting muscle health and gut health.

Preparation Time: 10 minutes

3: Turkey and Vegetable Stir-Fry

Ingredients:

- 4 oz cooked turkey breast, sliced
- 1 cup mixed vegetables (such as bell peppers, broccoli, carrots, and snap peas), sliced
- 1 tablespoon olive oil
- 2 cloves garlic, minced
- 1 teaspoon grated ginger
- 2 tablespoons low-sodium soy sauce
- 1 tablespoon rice vinegar
- 1 teaspoon honey or maple syrup (optional)
- 2 cups cooked brown rice or quinoa (for serving)
- Sesame seeds for garnish (optional)

Instructions:

- Heat olive oil in a large skillet or wok over medium-high heat.
- Add minced garlic and grated ginger to the skillet and sauté for 1-2 minutes until fragrant.
- Add sliced mixed vegetables to the skillet and stir-fry for 3-4 minutes until tender-crisp.
- Add sliced turkey breast to the skillet and stir-fry for another 2-3 minutes until heated through.
- In a small bowl, whisk together low-sodium soy sauce, rice vinegar, and honey or maple syrup (if using) to make the sauce.
- Pour the sauce over the turkey and vegetable mixture in the skillet.
- Stir well to coat evenly and cook for an additional 1-2 minutes.
- Remove the skillet from heat.
- Serve the turkey and vegetable stir-fry over cooked brown rice or quinoa.
- Optional: Garnish with sesame seeds for added flavor and texture.

Health Benefits:

- Turkey breast is a lean source of protein, supporting muscle health and satiety.
- Mixed vegetables offer vitamins, minerals, and antioxidants, promoting immune function and overall health.
- Brown rice or quinoa provides fiber and complex carbohydrates for sustained energy levels and digestive health.
- Olive oil offers heart-healthy fats and anti-inflammatory properties, contributing to cardiovascular health.

Preparation Time: 20 minutes

4: Lentil and Vegetable Soup

Ingredients:

- 1/2 cup dried green lentils, rinsed and drained
- 4 cups low-sodium vegetable broth
- 1 cup diced carrots
- 1 cup diced celery
- 1 cup diced onions

- 2 cloves garlic, minced
- 1 teaspoon dried thyme
- 1 bay leaf
- Salt and pepper to taste
- Fresh parsley for garnish (optional)

Instructions:

- In a large pot, combine dried green lentils, low-sodium vegetable broth, diced carrots, diced celery, diced onions, minced garlic, dried thyme, and bay leaf.
- Bring the mixture to a boil over medium-high heat.
- Reduce the heat to low, cover, and simmer for 20-25 minutes until the lentils and vegetables are tender.
- Season the soup with salt and pepper to taste.
- Remove the bay leaf from the soup.
- Ladle the lentil and vegetable soup into bowls.
- Optional: Garnish with fresh parsley for added flavor and presentation.
- Serve hot.

Health Benefits:

- Lentils are a good source of protein, fiber, and essential nutrients like iron and folate, supporting muscle health, digestion, and energy levels.
- Vegetables like carrots, celery, and onions provide vitamins, minerals, and antioxidants, promoting immune function and overall health.
- Vegetable broth adds flavor and hydration without added sodium, supporting kidney health and reducing the risk of hypertension.

Preparation Time: 30 minutes

5: Chicken and Quinoa Salad

Ingredients:

- 4 oz cooked chicken breast, diced
- 1/2 cup cooked quinoa
- 1 cup mixed greens (such as spinach, kale, and arugula)
- 1/4 cup cherry tomatoes, halved
- 1/4 cup diced cucumber
- 2 tablespoons diced red onion

- 1 tablespoon chopped fresh basil
- 1 tablespoon olive oil
- 1 tablespoon balsamic vinegar
- Salt and pepper to taste

Instructions:

- In a large bowl, combine diced chicken breast, cooked quinoa, mixed greens, cherry tomatoes, diced cucumber, diced red onion, and chopped fresh basil.
- In a small bowl, whisk together olive oil, balsamic vinegar, salt, and pepper to make the dressing.
- Pour the dressing over the salad ingredients in the large bowl.
- Toss gently to coat evenly.
- Divide the chicken and quinoa salad into serving bowls.
- Serve immediately.

Health Benefits:

- Chicken breast is a lean source of protein, supporting muscle health and satiety.

- Quinoa provides protein, fiber, and essential nutrients like iron and magnesium, promoting muscle health, digestion, and energy levels.
- Mixed greens, cherry tomatoes, cucumber, and red onion are rich in vitamins, minerals, and antioxidants, supporting immune function and overall health.
- Olive oil and balsamic vinegar offer heart-healthy fats and anti-inflammatory properties, contributing to cardiovascular health.

Preparation Time: 20 minutes

6: Tuna Salad Stuffed Bell Peppers

Ingredients:

- 2 large bell peppers (any color), halved and seeds removed
- 1 can (5 oz) tuna in water, drained
- 1/4 cup diced celery
- 1/4 cup diced red onion
- 2 tablespoons chopped fresh parsley
- 2 tablespoons plain Greek yogurt
- 1 tablespoon lemon juice

- Salt and pepper to taste
- Optional: sliced avocado for garnish

Instructions:

- Preheat the oven to 375°F (190°C).
- Place the halved bell peppers in a baking dish, cut side up.
- In a large bowl, combine drained tuna, diced celery, diced red onion, chopped fresh parsley, Greek yogurt, lemon juice, salt, and pepper.
- Mix well to combine all ingredients.
- Spoon the tuna salad mixture evenly into the bell pepper halves.
- Cover the baking dish with aluminum foil.
- Bake in the preheated oven for 20-25 minutes until the bell peppers are tender.
- Remove the foil and continue baking for an additional 5 minutes until the tops are lightly golden.
- Optional: Garnish with sliced avocado before serving.

Health Benefits:

- Bell peppers are rich in vitamins, minerals, and antioxidants, supporting immune function and overall health.
- Tuna is a good source of protein and omega-3 fatty acids, promoting muscle health, heart health, and brain function.
- Celery, red onion, and parsley offer additional vitamins, minerals, and antioxidants, contributing to digestive health, immune function, and detoxification.
- Greek yogurt provides protein and probiotics, supporting muscle health and gut health.

Preparation Time: 30 minutes

7: Mediterranean Chickpea Salad

Ingredients:

- 1 can (15 oz) chickpeas, rinsed and drained
- 1 cup diced cucumber
- 1 cup cherry tomatoes, halved
- 1/4 cup diced red onion

- 1/4 cup chopped fresh parsley
- 2 tablespoons chopped fresh mint
- 2 tablespoons extra virgin olive oil
- 1 tablespoon lemon juice
- 1 clove garlic, minced
- Salt and pepper to taste
- Optional: crumbled feta cheese for garnish

Instructions:

- In a large bowl, combine chickpeas, diced cucumber, cherry tomatoes, diced red onion, chopped fresh parsley, and chopped fresh mint.
- In a small bowl, whisk together extra virgin olive oil, lemon juice, minced garlic, salt, and pepper to make the dressing.
- Pour the dressing over the chickpea salad and toss gently to coat evenly.
- Optional: Sprinkle crumbled feta cheese on top for added flavor.
- Serve immediately or refrigerate until ready to eat.

Health Benefits:

- Chickpeas are rich in protein, fiber, and essential nutrients like iron and folate, promoting muscle health, digestion, and energy levels.
- Cucumber, cherry tomatoes, red onion, parsley, and mint offer vitamins, minerals, and antioxidants, supporting immune function and overall health.
- Extra virgin olive oil provides heart-healthy fats and anti-inflammatory properties, contributing to cardiovascular health and reduced inflammation.

Preparation Time: 15 minutes

8: Veggie and Hummus Wrap

Ingredients:

- 1 whole-grain tortilla
- 2 tablespoons hummus
- 1/4 cup shredded carrots
- 1/4 cup sliced cucumber
- 1/4 cup shredded lettuce
- 2 tablespoons diced red bell pepper
- 2 tablespoons diced avocado

- Salt and pepper to taste

Instructions:

- Spread hummus evenly over the whole-grain tortilla.
- Layer shredded carrots, sliced cucumber, shredded lettuce, diced red bell pepper, and diced avocado on top of the hummus.
- Season with salt and pepper to taste.
- Roll up the tortilla tightly to form a wrap.
- Optional: Secure the wrap with toothpicks or cut it in half for easier handling.
- Serve immediately or pack it for a convenient on-the-go lunch.

Health Benefits:

- Hummus offers plant-based protein, fiber, and healthy fats, supporting muscle health, satiety, and heart health.
- Vegetables like carrots, cucumber, lettuce, red bell pepper, and avocado provide vitamins, minerals, and antioxidants, promoting immune function, digestion, and overall health.

- Whole-grain tortillas provide fiber and complex carbohydrates for sustained energy levels and digestive health.

Preparation Time: 10 minutes

9: Veggie and Bean Quesadillas

Ingredients:

- 2 whole-grain tortillas
- 1/2 cup cooked black beans, drained and rinsed
- 1/2 cup diced bell peppers (any color)
- 1/4 cup diced red onion
- 1/4 cup corn kernels (fresh, frozen, or canned)
- 1/2 cup shredded low-fat cheese (such as cheddar or Monterey Jack)
- 1 tablespoon olive oil
- Salt and pepper to taste
- Optional toppings: salsa, Greek yogurt, sliced avocado

Instructions:

- Heat olive oil in a large skillet over medium heat.

- Add diced bell peppers and red onion to the skillet and sauté until softened, about 3-4 minutes.
- Add corn kernels and cooked black beans to the skillet, and cook for another 2 minutes until heated through.
- Season the mixture with salt and pepper to taste.
- Remove the skillet from heat and set aside.
- Place one whole-grain tortilla in the skillet over medium heat.
- Spread half of the shredded cheese evenly over the tortilla.
- Spoon half of the veggie and bean mixture on one half of the tortilla.
- Fold the other half of the tortilla over the filling to form a half-moon shape.
- Press down gently with a spatula and cook for 2-3 minutes until the bottom is golden brown and crispy.
- Carefully flip the quesadilla and cook for another 2-3 minutes until the other side is golden brown and crispy.
- Remove the quesadilla from the skillet and repeat the process with the remaining tortilla and filling.

- Slice the quesadillas into wedges and serve hot with optional toppings like salsa, Greek yogurt, or sliced avocado.

Health Benefits:

- Black beans are rich in fiber, protein, and essential nutrients like folate and magnesium, promoting digestive health, muscle health, and energy levels.
- Bell peppers, red onion, and corn offer vitamins, minerals, and antioxidants, supporting immune function and overall health.
- Whole-grain tortillas provide fiber and complex carbohydrates for sustained energy levels and digestive health.
- Low-fat cheese adds calcium and protein, contributing to bone health and satiety.

Preparation Time: 20 minutes

10: Spinach and Lentil Salad

Ingredients:

- 2 cups baby spinach leaves
- 1/2 cup cooked green lentils

- 1/4 cup diced cucumber
- 1/4 cup diced tomatoes
- 2 tablespoons diced red onion
- 2 tablespoons crumbled feta cheese
- 1 tablespoon chopped fresh dill
- 1 tablespoon extra virgin olive oil
- 1 tablespoon balsamic vinegar
- Salt and pepper to taste

Instructions:

- In a large bowl, combine baby spinach leaves, cooked green lentils, diced cucumber, diced tomatoes, diced red onion, crumbled feta cheese, and chopped fresh dill.
- In a small bowl, whisk together extra virgin olive oil, balsamic vinegar, salt, and pepper to make the dressing.
- Pour the dressing over the salad and toss gently to coat evenly.
- Divide the spinach and lentil salad into serving bowls.
- Serve immediately.

Health Benefits:

- Spinach is rich in vitamins, minerals, and antioxidants, supporting immune function and overall health.
- Green lentils provide protein, fiber, and essential nutrients like iron and folate, promoting muscle health, digestion, and energy levels.
- Cucumber, tomatoes, and red onion offer additional vitamins, minerals, and antioxidants, contributing to hydration, immune function, and digestive health.
- Feta cheese adds calcium and protein, contributing to bone health and satiety.

Preparation Time: 15 minutes

Kidney Disease Dinner Recipes for Women

1: Baked Salmon with Asparagus

Ingredients:

- 2 salmon fillets (4-6 oz each)
- 1 bunch asparagus, trimmed
- 2 tablespoons olive oil
- 2 cloves garlic, minced

- 1 teaspoon lemon zest
- 1 tablespoon lemon juice
- Salt and pepper to taste
- Fresh dill for garnish (optional)

Instructions:

- Preheat the oven to 400°F (200°C).
- Place the asparagus spears on a baking sheet and drizzle with 1 tablespoon of olive oil. Season with salt and pepper to taste.
- In a small bowl, mix together minced garlic, lemon zest, lemon juice, and the remaining tablespoon of olive oil.
- Place the salmon fillets on the baking sheet alongside the asparagus. Brush the salmon fillets with the garlic-lemon mixture.
- Bake in the preheated oven for 12-15 minutes, or until the salmon is cooked through and flakes easily with a fork.
- Remove from the oven and garnish with fresh dill, if desired.
- Serve the baked salmon with asparagus hot.

Health Benefits:

- Salmon is rich in omega-3 fatty acids, which are beneficial for heart health and reducing inflammation.
- Asparagus is a low-potassium vegetable that is high in fiber, folate, and vitamins A, C, and K.
- Olive oil contains heart-healthy monounsaturated fats and antioxidants that can reduce the risk of chronic diseases.
- Garlic has anti-inflammatory and immune-boosting properties.

Preparation Time: 20 minutes

2: Turkey and Vegetable Stir-Fry

Ingredients:

- 8 oz ground turkey
- 2 cups mixed vegetables (such as bell peppers, broccoli, carrots, and snap peas), sliced
- 2 cloves garlic, minced
- 2 tablespoons low-sodium soy sauce
- 1 tablespoon sesame oil

- 1 tablespoon rice vinegar
- 1 tablespoon honey or maple syrup (optional)
- Cooked brown rice or quinoa for serving

Instructions:

- Heat sesame oil in a large skillet or wok over medium heat.
- Add minced garlic to the skillet and sauté for 1-2 minutes until fragrant.
- Add ground turkey to the skillet and cook until browned, breaking it apart with a spoon.
- Add mixed vegetables to the skillet and stir-fry for 3-4 minutes until tender-crisp.
- In a small bowl, whisk together low-sodium soy sauce, rice vinegar, and honey or maple syrup (if using) to make the sauce.
- Pour the sauce over the turkey and vegetable mixture in the skillet.
- Stir well to coat evenly and cook for an additional 1-2 minutes.
- Remove from heat and serve the turkey and vegetable stir-fry over cooked brown rice or quinoa.

Health Benefits:

- Ground turkey is a lean source of protein that is lower in saturated fat compared to red meat.
- Mixed vegetables provide essential nutrients, vitamins, and minerals that support overall health and well-being.
- Brown rice or quinoa is a whole grain that is high in fiber and complex carbohydrates, providing sustained energy and promoting digestive health.
- Sesame oil contains healthy fats and antioxidants that can benefit heart health and reduce inflammation.

Preparation Time: 25 minutes

3: Veggie and Lentil Soup

Ingredients:

- 1 cup dried green or brown lentils, rinsed and drained
- 4 cups low-sodium vegetable broth
- 1 cup diced carrots
- 1 cup diced celery
- 1 cup diced onions
- 2 cloves garlic, minced

- 1 teaspoon dried thyme
- 1 bay leaf
- Salt and pepper to taste
- Fresh parsley for garnish (optional)

Instructions:

- In a large pot, combine dried lentils, low-sodium vegetable broth, diced carrots, diced celery, diced onions, minced garlic, dried thyme, and bay leaf.
- Bring the mixture to a boil over medium-high heat.
- Reduce the heat to low, cover, and simmer for 30-35 minutes until the lentils and vegetables are tender.
- Season the soup with salt and pepper to taste.
- Remove the bay leaf from the soup.
- Ladle the veggie and lentil soup into bowls.
- Garnish with fresh parsley for added flavor and presentation.
- Serve hot.

Health Benefits:

- Lentils are a good source of plant-based protein, fiber, and essential nutrients like iron and folate,

- promoting muscle health, digestion, and energy levels.
- Vegetables like carrots, celery, onions, and garlic provide vitamins, minerals, and antioxidants, supporting immune function, digestion, and overall health.
- Vegetable broth adds flavor and hydration without added sodium, supporting kidney health and reducing the risk of hypertension.

Preparation Time: 40 minutes

4: Grilled Chicken with Roasted Vegetables

Ingredients:

- 2 chicken breasts
- 2 cups mixed vegetables (such as bell peppers, zucchini, cherry tomatoes, and red onion), cut into bite-sized pieces
- 2 tablespoons olive oil
- 2 cloves garlic, minced
- 1 teaspoon dried Italian herbs (such as oregano, basil, and thyme)
- Salt and pepper to taste

- Lemon wedges for serving (optional)

Instructions:

- Preheat the grill to medium-high heat.
- In a large bowl, toss the mixed vegetables with olive oil, minced garlic, dried Italian herbs, salt, and pepper until evenly coated.
- Season the chicken breasts with salt and pepper on both sides.
- Place the chicken breasts on the grill and cook for 6-8 minutes per side, or until cooked through and no longer pink in the center.
- Meanwhile, spread the seasoned mixed vegetables in a single layer on a baking sheet.
- Place the baking sheet on the grill and cook the vegetables for 8-10 minutes, or until tender and lightly charred, stirring occasionally.
- Remove the chicken breasts and roasted vegetables from the grill.
- Serve the grilled chicken with roasted vegetables hot, with lemon wedges on the side for squeezing over the dish if desired.

Health Benefits:

- Chicken breast is a lean source of protein, promoting muscle health and satiety.
- Mixed vegetables offer a variety of vitamins, minerals, and antioxidants, supporting immune function, digestion, and overall health.
- Olive oil provides heart-healthy fats and anti-inflammatory properties, contributing to cardiovascular health.
- Grilling is a healthy cooking method that preserves the nutritional value of the ingredients while imparting a delicious smoky flavor.

Preparation Time: 25 minutes

5: Quinoa Stuffed Bell Peppers

Ingredients:

- 4 large bell peppers (any color), halved and seeds removed
- 1 cup cooked quinoa
- 1 can (15 oz) black beans, rinsed and drained
- 1 cup diced tomatoes

- 1/2 cup diced onions
- 1/2 cup corn kernels (fresh, frozen, or canned)
- 1 teaspoon chili powder
- 1/2 teaspoon cumin
- Salt and pepper to taste
- 1/2 cup shredded low-fat cheese (such as cheddar or Monterey Jack)
- Fresh cilantro for garnish (optional)

Instructions:

- Preheat the oven to 375°F (190°C).
- Place the halved bell peppers in a baking dish, cut side up.
- In a large bowl, combine cooked quinoa, black beans, diced tomatoes, diced onions, corn kernels, chili powder, cumin, salt, and pepper.
- Spoon the quinoa mixture evenly into the bell pepper halves.
- Cover the baking dish with aluminum foil.
- Bake in the preheated oven for 30-35 minutes, or until the bell peppers are tender.

- Remove the foil and sprinkle shredded cheese on top of each stuffed bell pepper.
- Return to the oven and bake for an additional 5 minutes, or until the cheese is melted and bubbly.
- Remove from the oven and garnish with fresh cilantro, if desired.
- Serve hot.

Health Benefits:

- Bell peppers are low in potassium and rich in vitamins A and C, supporting immune function and eye health.
- Quinoa is a complete protein and a good source of fiber, promoting muscle health, satiety, and digestive health.
- Black beans provide protein, fiber, and essential nutrients like iron and folate, supporting muscle health, digestion, and energy levels.
- Tomatoes are rich in vitamins, minerals, and antioxidants, offering numerous health benefits including improved heart health and reduced inflammation.

Preparation Time: 45 minutes

6: Veggie Stir-Fry with Tofu

Ingredients:

- 1 block (14 oz) firm tofu, drained and pressed
- 2 tablespoons low-sodium soy sauce
- 1 tablespoon sesame oil
- 2 cloves garlic, minced
- 1 teaspoon grated ginger
- 2 cups mixed vegetables (such as broccoli, bell peppers, snap peas, and carrots), sliced
- Cooked brown rice or quinoa for serving
- Sesame seeds for garnish (optional)
- Sliced green onions for garnish (optional)

Instructions:

- Cut the pressed tofu into cubes and place them in a bowl.
- In a small bowl, whisk together low-sodium soy sauce, sesame oil, minced garlic, and grated ginger to make the marinade.

- Pour the marinade over the tofu cubes and toss gently to coat evenly. Let marinate for 10-15 minutes.
- Heat a large skillet or wok over medium-high heat.
- Add the marinated tofu cubes to the skillet and cook for 5-6 minutes, stirring occasionally, until browned and crispy.
- Remove the tofu from the skillet and set aside.
- In the same skillet, add mixed vegetables and stir-fry for 4-5 minutes until tender-crisp.
- Return the tofu to the skillet and toss with the vegetables to combine.
- Serve the veggie stir-fry with tofu over cooked brown rice or quinoa.
- Garnish with sesame seeds and sliced green onions, if desired.
- Serve hot.

Health Benefits:

- Tofu is a plant-based protein that is low in saturated fat and cholesterol, making it heart-healthy and kidney-friendly.

- Mixed vegetables provide a variety of vitamins, minerals, and antioxidants, supporting immune function, digestion, and overall health.
- Brown rice or quinoa offers fiber and complex carbohydrates for sustained energy levels and digestive health.
- Sesame oil adds flavor and heart-healthy fats, while garlic and ginger provide anti-inflammatory and immune-boosting properties.

Preparation Time: 30 minutes

7: Mediterranean Chicken Skewers with Greek Salad

Ingredients for Chicken Skewers:

- 2 boneless, skinless chicken breasts, cut into cubes
- 1 tablespoon olive oil
- 2 cloves garlic, minced
- 1 teaspoon dried oregano
- 1 teaspoon dried basil
- Salt and pepper to taste
- Wooden skewers, soaked in water for 30 minutes

Ingredients for Greek Salad:

- 2 cups mixed salad greens
- 1 cup cherry tomatoes, halved
- 1 cucumber, diced
- 1/4 cup diced red onion
- 1/4 cup crumbled feta cheese
- 2 tablespoons chopped Kalamata olives
- 1 tablespoon extra virgin olive oil
- 1 tablespoon lemon juice
- 1 teaspoon dried oregano
- Salt and pepper to taste

Instructions:

- In a bowl, combine olive oil, minced garlic, dried oregano, dried basil, salt, and pepper. Add chicken cubes and toss to coat. Marinate in the refrigerator for at least 30 minutes.
- Prehcat the grill or grill pan over medium-high heat. Thread marinated chicken onto soaked skewers.
- Grill chicken skewers for 6-8 minutes per side or until cooked through and lightly charred.

- In a large salad bowl, combine mixed greens, cherry tomatoes, cucumber, red onion, feta cheese, and Kalamata olives.
- In a small bowl, whisk together extra virgin olive oil, lemon juice, dried oregano, salt, and pepper to make the dressing.
- Drizzle the dressing over the Greek salad and toss to coat evenly.
- Serve the grilled chicken skewers with Greek salad on the side.

Health Benefits:

- Chicken breast is a lean source of protein, promoting muscle health and satiety.
- Mediterranean herbs like oregano and basil add flavor and contain antioxidants that support overall health.
- Mixed greens, tomatoes, cucumber, red onion, and olives in the salad provide vitamins, minerals, and fiber, promoting digestive health and immune function.

- Olive oil offers heart-healthy monounsaturated fats and anti-inflammatory properties.

Preparation Time: 40 minutes

8: Lentil and Vegetable Curry

Ingredients:

- 1 cup dried green lentils, rinsed and drained
- 4 cups low-sodium vegetable broth
- 1 tablespoon olive oil
- 1 onion, diced
- 2 cloves garlic, minced
- 1 tablespoon grated ginger
- 1 tablespoon curry powder
- 1 teaspoon ground cumin
- 1 teaspoon ground turmeric
- 1 teaspoon paprika
- 1 can (14 oz) diced tomatoes
- 2 cups mixed vegetables (such as cauliflower, carrots, and bell peppers), diced
- Salt and pepper to taste
- Cooked brown rice for serving

- Fresh cilantro for garnish (optional)

Instructions:

- In a large pot, heat olive oil over medium heat. Add diced onion and cook until softened, about 5 minutes.
- Add minced garlic, grated ginger, curry powder, ground cumin, ground turmeric, and paprika to the pot. Stir well and cook for 1-2 minutes until fragrant.
- Add diced tomatoes (with their juices), mixed vegetables, dried green lentils, and vegetable broth to the pot. Stir to combine.
- Bring the mixture to a boil, then reduce the heat to low. Cover and simmer for 25-30 minutes, or until the lentils and vegetables are tender.
- Season the curry with salt and pepper to taste.
- Serve the lentil and vegetable curry hot over cooked brown rice.
- Garnish with fresh cilantro, if desired.

Health Benefits:

- Lentils are a good source of plant-based protein, fiber, and essential nutrients like iron and folate,

promoting muscle health, digestion, and energy levels.
- Mixed vegetables provide vitamins, minerals, and antioxidants, supporting immune function, digestion, and overall health.
- Spices like curry powder, cumin, turmeric, and paprika offer anti-inflammatory and immune-boosting properties.
- Brown rice is a whole grain that provides fiber and complex carbohydrates for sustained energy levels and digestive health.

Preparation Time: 45 minutes

9: Baked Cod with Lemon Herb Crust

Ingredients:

- 4 cod fillets (about 6 oz each)
- 2 tablespoons olive oil
- 2 cloves garlic, minced
- Zest of 1 lemon
- 1 tablespoon chopped fresh parsley
- 1 tablespoon chopped fresh dill
- Salt and pepper to taste

- Lemon wedges for serving
- Steamed green beans or broccoli for serving

Instructions:

- Preheat the oven to 400°F (200°C).
- In a small bowl, mix together olive oil, minced garlic, lemon zest, chopped parsley, chopped dill, salt, and pepper.
- Place the cod fillets on a baking sheet lined with parchment paper.
- Brush the lemon herb mixture evenly over the top of each cod fillet.
- Bake in the preheated oven for 12-15 minutes, or until the fish flakes easily with a fork and is opaque in the center.
- Remove from the oven and serve hot with lemon wedges on the side.
- Serve with steamed green beans or broccoli for a complete meal.

Health Benefits:

- Cod is a lean source of protein that is low in saturated fat and rich in omega-3 fatty acids, which are beneficial for heart health and reducing inflammation.
- Olive oil provides heart-healthy monounsaturated fats and antioxidants that can reduce the risk of chronic diseases.
- Garlic and herbs like parsley and dill add flavor and contain antioxidants that support overall health.
- Green beans and broccoli are low-potassium vegetables that are high in fiber, vitamins, and minerals, promoting digestive health and immune function.

Preparation Time: 20 minutes

10: Turkey Meatballs with Marinara Sauce

Ingredients for Turkey Meatballs:

- 1 lb lean ground turkey
- 1/4 cup breadcrumbs (gluten-free if needed)
- 1/4 cup grated Parmesan cheese

- 1/4 cup chopped fresh parsley
- 1 egg, beaten
- 2 cloves garlic, minced
- 1/2 teaspoon dried oregano
- Salt and pepper to taste

Ingredients for Marinara Sauce:

- 1 can (14 oz) crushed tomatoes
- 2 cloves garlic, minced
- 1 teaspoon dried basil
- 1 teaspoon dried oregano
- Salt and pepper to taste

Instructions:

- Preheat the oven to 375°F (190°C).
- In a large bowl, combine ground turkey, breadcrumbs, grated Parmesan cheese, chopped parsley, beaten egg, minced garlic, dried oregano, salt, and pepper. Mix until well combined.
- Shape the mixture into meatballs, about 1 inch in diameter, and place them on a baking sheet lined with parchment paper.

- Bake in the preheated oven for 20-25 minutes, or until the meatballs are cooked through and browned on the outside.
- While the meatballs are baking, prepare the marinara sauce. In a saucepan, combine crushed tomatoes, minced garlic, dried basil, dried oregano, salt, and pepper. Cook over medium heat for 10-15 minutes, stirring occasionally.
- Once the meatballs are cooked, transfer them to the saucepan with the marinara sauce. Gently stir to coat the meatballs with the sauce.
- Serve the turkey meatballs with marinara sauce hot, over cooked whole-grain pasta or zucchini noodles.

Health Benefits:

- Lean ground turkey is a good source of protein that is lower in saturated fat compared to red meat, promoting muscle health and satiety.
- Breadcrumbs and Parmesan cheese add texture and flavor to the meatballs without excess sodium.

- Fresh herbs like parsley, garlic, basil, and oregano provide antioxidants and anti-inflammatory properties.
- Crushed tomatoes are rich in vitamins, minerals, and antioxidants, supporting immune function and overall health.

Preparation Time: 45 minutes

Kidney Disease Snacks Recipes for Women

1: Avocado and White Bean Dip with Veggie Sticks

Ingredients for Avocado and White Bean Dip:

- 1 ripe avocado, peeled and pitted
- 1 can (15 oz) white beans, drained and rinsed
- 2 tablespoons fresh lemon juice
- 1 clove garlic, minced
- 2 tablespoons chopped fresh cilantro
- Salt and pepper to taste

Ingredients for Veggie Sticks:

- Assorted vegetables (carrot sticks, cucumber slices, bell pepper strips, celery sticks, etc.)

Instructions:

- In a food processor or blender, combine ripe avocado, white beans, fresh lemon juice, minced garlic, chopped cilantro, salt, and pepper.
- Blend until smooth and creamy, adding a splash of water if needed to reach the desired consistency.
- Transfer the avocado and white bean dip to a serving bowl.
- Prepare assorted vegetables by washing, peeling, and cutting them into sticks, slices, or strips.
- Arrange the veggie sticks around the dip bowl for serving.
- Enjoy the avocado and white bean dip with veggie sticks as a nutritious snack.

Health Benefits:

- Avocado is a heart-healthy fruit rich in monounsaturated fats, fiber, and vitamins.

- White beans are a good source of plant-based protein, fiber, and essential nutrients like iron and folate, promoting muscle health, digestion, and energy levels.
- Assorted vegetables provide vitamins, minerals, and antioxidants, supporting immune function, digestion, and overall health.
- This snack is low in sodium and saturated fat, making it suitable for individuals with kidney disease.

Preparation Time: 10 minutes

2: Greek Yogurt Parfait with Berries and Almonds

Ingredients:

- 1 cup plain Greek yogurt
- 1/2 cup mixed berries (such as strawberries, blueberries, and raspberries)
- 2 tablespoons slivered almonds
- 1 tablespoon honey or maple syrup (optional)
- Dash of cinnamon (optional)

Instructions:

- In a serving glass or bowl, layer plain Greek yogurt with mixed berries and slivered almonds.
- Drizzle honey or maple syrup over the yogurt and berries if desired, for added sweetness.
- Sprinkle a dash of cinnamon on top for extra flavor, if desired.
- Repeat the layering process until all ingredients are used up or until the serving container is filled.
- Serve the Greek yogurt parfait immediately or refrigerate until ready to eat.

Health Benefits:

- Greek yogurt is high in protein and low in carbohydrates, making it a satisfying snack that can help stabilize blood sugar levels and promote satiety.
- Berries are low in calories and high in fiber, vitamins, and antioxidants, supporting immune function and overall health.
- Almonds are a good source of healthy fats, protein, and fiber, providing energy and promoting heart health.

- This snack is rich in calcium, probiotics, and essential nutrients, making it beneficial for bone health, digestion, and gut health.

Preparation Time: 5 minutes

3: Hummus with Whole Grain Pita Chips

Ingredients for Hummus:

- 1 can (15 oz) chickpeas, drained and rinsed
- 2 tablespoons tahini (sesame seed paste)
- 2 cloves garlic, minced
- 2 tablespoons fresh lemon juice
- 2 tablespoons olive oil
- 1/2 teaspoon ground cumin
- Salt and pepper to taste
- Water (as needed for desired consistency)

Ingredients for Whole Grain Pita Chips:

- 2 whole grain pita bread rounds
- 1 tablespoon olive oil
- 1/2 teaspoon garlic powder
- 1/2 teaspoon paprika
- Salt to taste

Instructions:

- In a food processor, combine chickpeas, tahini, minced garlic, fresh lemon juice, olive oil, ground cumin, salt, and pepper.
- Blend until smooth, adding water as needed to reach the desired consistency.
- Transfer the hummus to a serving bowl and set aside.
- Preheat the oven to 375°F (190°C).
- Cut each whole grain pita bread round into triangles or wedges.
- In a small bowl, mix together olive oil, garlic powder, paprika, and salt.
- Place the pita chips on a baking sheet and brush them with the olive oil mixture on both sides.
- Bake in the preheated oven for 10-12 minutes, or until the pita chips are golden brown and crispy.
- Remove from the oven and let cool slightly before serving.
- Serve the hummus with whole grain pita chips for dipping.

Health Benefits:

- Chickpeas are rich in fiber, protein, and essential nutrients like iron and folate, promoting digestive health, muscle health, and energy levels.
- Tahini is a good source of healthy fats, protein, and minerals like calcium and magnesium, supporting bone health and heart health.
- Whole grain pita bread provides fiber and complex carbohydrates for sustained energy levels and digestive health.
- Olive oil contains heart-healthy monounsaturated fats and antioxidants that can reduce the risk of chronic diseases.

Preparation Time: 20 minutes

4: Cottage Cheese with Sliced Peaches and Almonds

Ingredients:

- 1/2 cup low-fat cottage cheese
- 1 ripe peach, sliced
- 2 tablespoons slivered almonds

- 1 teaspoon honey (optional)

Instructions:

- In a serving bowl, spoon low-fat cottage cheese.
- Arrange sliced peaches on top of the cottage cheese.
- Sprinkle slivered almonds over the peaches.
- Drizzle honey over the top for added sweetness, if desired.
- Serve the cottage cheese with sliced peaches and almonds immediately.

Health Benefits:

- Low-fat cottage cheese is a good source of protein and calcium, promoting muscle health and bone health.
- Peaches are low in calories and high in fiber, vitamins, and antioxidants, supporting immune function, digestion, and overall health.
- Almonds are rich in healthy fats, protein, and fiber, providing energy and promoting heart health.
- This snack is low in sodium and saturated fat, making it suitable for individuals with kidney disease.

Preparation Time: 5 minutes

5: Tuna Salad Stuffed Cucumber Boats

Ingredients:

- 1 can (5 oz) tuna in water, drained
- 2 tablespoons plain Greek yogurt
- 1 tablespoon chopped fresh dill
- 1 tablespoon lemon juice
- Salt and pepper to taste
- 2 large cucumbers
- Cherry tomatoes for garnish (optional)

Instructions:

- In a mixing bowl, combine drained tuna, plain Greek yogurt, chopped fresh dill, lemon juice, salt, and pepper. Mix until well combined.
- Cut the cucumbers in half lengthwise and scoop out the seeds with a spoon to create "boats."
- Divide the tuna salad mixture evenly among the cucumber boats, filling each one.
- Garnish with cherry tomatoes, if desired, for added color and flavor.

- Serve the tuna salad stuffed cucumber boats immediately or refrigerate until ready to eat.

Health Benefits:

- Tuna is a lean source of protein and omega-3 fatty acids, which are beneficial for heart health and reducing inflammation.
- Greek yogurt provides additional protein and probiotics, supporting digestive health and immune function.
- Cucumbers are low in calories and high in water content, helping to hydrate the body and promote satiety.
- This snack is low in carbohydrates and sodium, making it suitable for individuals with kidney disease.

Preparation Time: 10 minutes

6: Rice Cake with Almond Butter and Banana Slices

Ingredients:

- 1 rice cake (preferably low-sodium)

- 1 tablespoon almond butter
- 1/2 ripe banana, sliced
- Drizzle of honey (optional)
- Pinch of cinnamon (optional)

Instructions:

- Spread almond butter evenly on top of the rice cake.
- Arrange banana slices on top of the almond butter.
- Drizzle with honey and sprinkle with cinnamon, if desired, for added sweetness and flavor.
- Serve the rice cake with almond butter and banana slices immediately.

Health Benefits:

- Rice cakes are low in calories and carbohydrates, providing a crunchy base for toppings without excess sodium.
- Almond butter is a good source of healthy fats, protein, and fiber, providing sustained energy and promoting heart health.

- Bananas are rich in potassium, vitamins, and minerals, supporting muscle function, digestion, and overall health.
- This snack is quick and easy to prepare, making it ideal for busy schedules and on-the-go snacking.

Preparation Time: 5 minutes

7: Edamame Hummus with Raw Veggie Dippers

Ingredients for Edamame Hummus:

- 1 cup shelled edamame (frozen and thawed)
- 2 tablespoons tahini (sesame seed paste)
- 2 tablespoons fresh lemon juice
- 1 clove garlic, minced
- 2 tablespoons olive oil
- Salt and pepper to taste
- Water (as needed for desired consistency)

Ingredients for Raw Veggie Dippers:

- Assorted raw vegetables (such as carrot sticks, cucumber slices, bell pepper strips, and snap peas)

Instructions:

- In a food processor or blender, combine shelled edamame, tahini, fresh lemon juice, minced garlic, olive oil, salt, and pepper.
- Blend until smooth, adding water as needed to reach the desired consistency.
- Transfer the edamame hummus to a serving bowl.
- Wash, peel, and cut assorted raw vegetables into sticks, slices, or strips for dipping.
- Arrange the raw veggie dippers around the hummus bowl for serving.
- Enjoy the edamame hummus with raw veggie dippers as a nutritious snack.

Health Benefits:

- Edamame is a good source of plant-based protein, fiber, and essential nutrients like iron and folate, promoting muscle health, digestion, and energy levels.
- Tahini is rich in healthy fats, protein, and minerals like calcium and magnesium, supporting bone health and heart health.

- Assorted raw vegetables provide vitamins, minerals, and antioxidants, supporting immune function, digestion, and overall health.
- This snack is low in sodium and saturated fat, making it suitable for individuals with kidney disease.

Preparation Time: 10 minutes

8: Apple Slices with Peanut Butter and Chia Seeds

Ingredients:

- 1 medium apple, cored and sliced
- 2 tablespoons natural peanut butter (unsweetened)
- 1 tablespoon chia seeds

Instructions:

- Core and slice the apple into thin rounds or wedges.
- Spread natural peanut butter on each apple slice.
- Sprinkle chia seeds over the peanut butter for added texture and nutrition.
- Serve the apple slices with peanut butter and chia seeds immediately.

Health Benefits:

- Apples are low in calories and high in fiber, vitamins, and antioxidants, supporting digestive health, heart health, and immune function.
- Natural peanut butter is a good source of healthy fats, protein, and fiber, providing energy and promoting satiety.
- Chia seeds are rich in omega-3 fatty acids, fiber, and antioxidants, supporting heart health, digestion, and overall wellness.
- This snack is quick, easy, and portable, making it ideal for busy schedules and on-the-go snacking.

Preparation Time: 5 minutes

9: Cucumber and Cottage Cheese Bites

Ingredients:

- 1 cucumber
- 1/2 cup low-fat cottage cheese
- 1 tablespoon chopped fresh chives or dill
- Salt and pepper to taste

Instructions:

- Wash the cucumber and slice it into rounds, about 1/2 inch thick.
- Using a small spoon or melon baller, scoop out a small indentation in the center of each cucumber round to create a cup.
- In a small bowl, mix together the low-fat cottage cheese, chopped fresh chives or dill, salt, and pepper.
- Spoon a small amount of the cottage cheese mixture into each cucumber cup.
- Garnish with additional chopped chives or dill, if desired.
- Serve the cucumber and cottage cheese bites immediately or refrigerate until ready to eat.

Health Benefits:

- Cucumbers are low in calories and high in water content, helping to hydrate the body and promote satiety.
- Low-fat cottage cheese is a good source of protein and calcium, supporting muscle health and bone health.

- Fresh herbs like chives or dill add flavor and contain antioxidants that support overall health.
- This snack is low in carbohydrates and sodium, making it suitable for individuals with kidney disease.

Preparation Time: 10 minutes

10: Banana and Walnut Oat Bites

Ingredients:

- 1 ripe banana
- 1/2 cup rolled oats
- 1/4 cup chopped walnuts
- 1 tablespoon honey or maple syrup (optional)
- 1/2 teaspoon ground cinnamon
- Pinch of salt

Instructions:

- Preheat the oven to 350°F (175°C). Line a baking sheet with parchment paper.
- In a mixing bowl, mash the ripe banana with a fork until smooth.

- Add rolled oats, chopped walnuts, honey or maple syrup (if using), ground cinnamon, and a pinch of salt to the bowl. Stir until well combined.
- Using a tablespoon or cookie scoop, portion the mixture and roll it into small balls.
- Place the oat bites onto the prepared baking sheet, spacing them apart.
- Flatten each oat bite slightly with the back of a spoon or your fingers.
- Bake in the preheated oven for 12-15 minutes, or until the oat bites are golden brown and firm.
- Remove from the oven and let cool on the baking sheet for a few minutes before transferring to a wire rack to cool completely.
- Serve the banana and walnut oat bites as a nutritious snack.

Health Benefits:

- Bananas are rich in potassium, vitamins, and minerals, supporting muscle function, digestion, and overall health.

- Rolled oats provide fiber, complex carbohydrates, and essential nutrients, promoting digestive health and sustained energy levels.
- Walnuts are high in healthy fats, protein, and antioxidants, supporting heart health, brain health, and overall wellness.
- This snack is naturally sweetened with fruit and optional honey or maple syrup, making it a healthier alternative to store-bought snacks.

Preparation Time: 20 minutes

CONCLUSION

The Kidney Disease Diet Cookbook for Women offers a comprehensive and empowering resource tailored specifically to the unique dietary needs of women managing kidney disease.

Through a diverse array of flavorful recipes, meticulously crafted to align with renal health guidelines, this cookbook not only provides delicious meal options but also serves as a supportive companion on the journey to improved wellness.

By embracing the principles of kidney-friendly nutrition, women can take proactive steps towards managing their condition and optimizing their overall health and well-being.

From breakfast to dinner, and even snacks in between, each recipe is thoughtfully curated to prioritize nutrient-rich ingredients, promote balanced eating, and inspire culinary creativity.

Moreover, beyond its role as a cookbook, this resource serves as a beacon of education, offering valuable insights into the causes, symptoms, and risk factors associated with kidney disease in women.

Armed with knowledge and armed with flavorful, nourishing recipes, women are empowered to make informed choices and take charge of their health.

As women navigate the complexities of kidney disease, this cookbook stands as a steadfast ally, offering not just recipes, but also hope, inspiration, and the promise of a brighter, healthier future.

With each meal prepared, each bite savored, and each step taken towards wellness, women embark on a transformative journey towards improved kidney health and enhanced quality of life.

www.ingramcontent.com/pod-product-compliance
Lightning Source LLC
Chambersburg PA
CBHW050323230526
45471CB00005B/2322